BITS & BYTES

A GUIDE TO DIGITALLY TRACKING YOUR FOOD, FITNESS, AND HEALTH

Meagan F. Moyer MPH, RDN, LD
and the Academy of Nutrition and Dietetics

 **eat right.** Academy of Nutrition and Dietetics

Bits and Bytes: A Guide to Digitally Tracking Your Food, Fitness, and Health

ISBN 978-0-88091-492-5 print

ISBN 978-0-88091-493-2 eBook

Catalog Number 492517, 492517e

For more information on the Academy of Nutrition and Dietetics, visit www.eatright.org.

10   9   8   7   6   5   4   3   2   1

Library of Congress Cataloging-in-Publication Data

Names: Moyer, Meagan F. | Academy of Nutrition and Dietetics.

Title: Bits and bytes : a guide to digitally tracking your food, fitness, and health / Meagan Moyer MPH, RDN, LD and the Academy of Nutrition and Dietetics.

Description: Chicago : Academy of Nutrition and Dietetics, [2017] | Includes index.

Identifiers: LCCN 2016033088 (print) | LCCN 2016025588 (ebook) | ISBN 9780880914925 (print) | ISBN 9780880914932 (ebook)

Subjects: LCSH: Physical fitness. | Health--Computer network resources.

Classification: LCC RA781 .M69 2017 (print) | LCC RA781 (ebook) | DDC 613.7--dc23

LC record available at https://lccn.loc.gov/2016025588

CONTENTS

REVIEWERS

JILL KOHN, MS, RDN, LDN
Knowledge Center at the Academy of Nutrition and Dietetics
Chicago, IL

MARISA MOORE, MBA, RDN, LD
Spokesperson, Consultant, Speaker
Atlanta, GA

ABOUT
THE AUTHOR

MEAGAN F. MOYER, MPH, RDN, LD, is a registered dietitian nutritionist and member of the Academy of Nutrition and Dietetics. She is the Coordinator of Nutrition Services at the Emory Bariatric Center, a comprehensive, multidisciplinary weight management clinic in Atlanta, GA. Meagan is also a healthy cooking instructor at a local cooking school. With many years' experience in adult weight management, she has appeared in numerous media outlets as a nutrition expert, including local news shows, CNN, and WebMD. Meagan earned a master's degree in public health from Emory University and a bachelor of science degree in dietetics from Purdue University. Meagan enjoys running, dancing, and practicing yoga (using activity tracking devices, of course!). She lives in Atlanta, GA.

INTRODUCTION

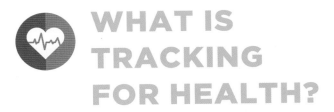

WHAT IS TRACKING FOR HEALTH?

Your sister logs the food she eats on a website. Your neighbor counts his steps using a fitness application, or "app," on his smartphone. Your aunt writes down her blood sugar levels to show her doctor. What do these people have in common? They all track for their health! Keeping track of key health habits, like what foods you eat, how often you exercise, how much water you drink, and how well you sleep, can make a big difference in improving your health.

Many people keep track of health habits. In 2012, the Pew Research Center asked 3,000 adults about their health-tracking habits. They found that 7 out of 10 people tracked health measures "for themselves or for a loved one." They also found the following:

- 60% tracked their weight, diet, or exercise routine; and
- 33% tracked important health numbers like blood pressure, blood sugar, and how many hours slept.

People track their health habits in many ways. The Pew Research Center study found the following:

- 49% kept track of progress "in their heads,"
- 34% recorded their progress in a notebook or journal, and

- 21% used technology like a website or an app on their phone.

(Note: While any kind of tracking can be helpful, keeping track of your eating and exercise habits only in your head might not be enough when trying to make a change or meet a goal.)

The survey also found that many people share the information they track with their doctor or other health experts, with their spouse or partner, with family members, and with friends. Sharing tracking data with other people helps with motivation and support. We will discuss this more in Chapter 3 and Chapter 6.

WHAT ARE DIGITAL HEALTH TOOLS?

Technology moves very fast. The way we use technology today is very different from the way we used it even just 5 years ago. Now more than ever, computers and cell phones are changing the way we communicate, learn, work, and play. Technology is changing the way we think about our health, too. Digital health-tracking tools are becoming more popular and include devices that are worn or carried (including cell phones). These devices are used to measure a person's health habits.

If you have a smartphone, tablet, or computer, you can use digital health tools. They are easy to use and can be inexpensive—in fact, many websites and apps are free. Wearable devices are more expensive than apps and websites, but they can tell you a lot more information. A list of popular websites, apps, and devices is included in Chapter 5.

WHAT ARE THE BENEFITS OF DIGITAL HEALTH TOOLS?

Why would you use digital tools to measure your health? You can use them to do the following:

- develop healthy habits, such as eating right or being physically active;
- manage your weight;
- help prevent or improve health conditions, such as diabetes, high blood pressure, or high cholesterol; and
- share information with your health care providers and get feedback on your health.

Many medical doctors, exercise specialists, and registered dietitian nutritionists (RDNs) use digital health tools with their clients. Health care providers are asking patients to track health details such as the symptoms they experience, the food they eat, and how often they exercise. Patients can receive better care from their health care providers when they share their health-tracking information. By sharing and tracking, patients take control of their own health.

You'll learn more about the benefits of using digital tools in Chapter 1.

HOW CAN THIS BOOK HELP ME?

This book will explain how digital health tracking can help you achieve your health and fitness goals. It will cover how to:

- get started with digital tracking,
- decide which health habits to track and why, and
- choose from among the many digital tracking tools available.

? DID YOU KNOW?

Leonardo Da Vinci is credited with conceptualizing the first pedometer!

Benjamin Franklin kept detailed journals on his mental health and personal growth.

You will read about RDNs who use digital tracking with their clients. You will also read success stories from people who track their own health habits. We welcome you to join the growing number of people who track for better health!

COMMON TERMS

Here are some common terms related to weight management and digital health tracking.

APPLICATION OR APP: a software program that performs a specific task (such as a game, a media player, or a map). Users download apps onto a desktop computer or onto a mobile device, such as a smartphone or tablet.

BODY MASS INDEX (BMI): the ratio of a person's weight to height. BMI is used to determine a person's risk for health conditions. In general, higher BMI numbers equal more risk for developing a weight-related health condition.

CALORIE: a unit of energy that comes from eating food and drinking beverages. Carbohydrates, protein, and fat in foods provide our bodies with calories.

DIGITAL HEALTH TRACKING: using technology, through websites, applications (apps), or other devices, to record habits with the goal of improving your health.

DOWNLOAD: putting an application or program onto your computer, smartphone, or tablet. Most applications and programs come from the Internet.

HEALTH DATA: pieces of information that can be used to analyze a health behavior or condition. Medical professionals use health data to make treatment recommendations. You can use health data from digital tracking to improve your health too.

SEARCH BOX: a rectangular box on a website or app in which you type in a word or phrase you want to look up.

SELF-MONITORING: keeping track of your own habits to keep or change those actions for the better.

SMARTPHONE: A cellular phone that performs many of the functions of a computer, typically having a touchscreen, Internet access, and an operating system that is able to run apps.

WEARABLE DEVICE OR WEARABLE TECHNOLOGY: a wireless device that is worn or carried by a person to track and record personal health data.

CHAPTER 1

IS DIGITAL TRACKING RIGHT FOR ME?

TRACKING CAN HELP anyone who wants to improve his or her health! It works because it helps people become more aware of their eating, exercise, and health-related habits. Some of the health concerns of trackers may include:

- overweight or obesity,
- reaching or maintaining a healthy weight,
- diabetes, or
- high blood pressure.

Of these, tracking to help lose weight is the most popular. Studies have shown that tracking helps people lose weight and keep it off. To meet their weight goals, many people who track regularly log the food they eat, how much exercise they do, and how much they weigh. There are three main ways to track these habits:

- paper records (pen and paper)
- tracking websites
- mobile devices (mobile phones and wearable physical activity devices)

This guide will focus on the last two ways to track: using websites and mobile devices. While losing weight may be the most popular reason to use digital tracking, once you decide to track, you can use it to help meet any of your health goals!

WHY SHOULD I GO DIGITAL?

Tracking is clearly helpful to those looking to manage their weight and improve their health. But does that mean you need to go digital? In the past, many people successfully met their health goals using pen and paper to track their food. This may have involved looking up foods in a calorie-counter book. Today, technology offers many features that can make tracking easier. It can create a more complete picture of your personal health data.

BENEFITS OF DIGITAL TRACKING

Why are more people turning to digital tracking? It offers many benefits that can help them reach their goals. Digital tracking is:

FAST. Once you get the hang of the technology, using digital trackers is quicker than using pen and paper. For example, many food trackers store your commonly eaten foods in a favorites list so you don't need to look them up every time. You can also copy entire meals from one day to the next with one or two clicks.

EASY. Digital trackers do the math for you. They automatically add up the calories you eat at each meal throughout the day. They can total the number of calories you burn during activity, too. At a glance, you can see where you stand in the balance of calories in and calories out.

CUSTOMIZED. Most fitness trackers use your specific information, such as your age, weight, level of activity, and other factors, to determine a realistic amount of calories you burn during activity and how many calories you should eat to reach your goals.

COMPREHENSIVE. With pen and paper, you may find it possible to track the basics, such as number of calories eaten, hours of sleep, minutes per type of activity, and so on. Digital tracking can do so much more. It calculates nutrients, which can help with weight management. Some tracking devices can tell you how often you wake during the night. They can measure your pace, mileage, and heart rate during physical activity.

These are just a few examples. Chapter 2 goes into more detail about the many features of tracking devices.

VISUAL. Digital trackers turn the data you enter into graphs and charts that help you better understand how to manage your weight. For example, food trackers can break down your daily intake into a pie chart to show you what percentage of your calories came from carbohydrates, fat, and protein. You can track your weight loss over time with a line graph—and watching that line go down is an encouraging sight!

FUN! Games, competitions, and rewards are built into many digital tracking tools. They can motivate you to stick to your goals, make your workouts more fun, and provide a community of like-minded supporters.

SHAREABLE. It's easy to share your tracking information and progress with your doctor and registered dietitian nutritionist (RDN). When they have this tracking information, they can easily make changes to their recommendations for you. Many RDNs encourage their clients to send them photos or records of what they eat, along with their food and exercise journals. Digital trackers make sharing this information easy!

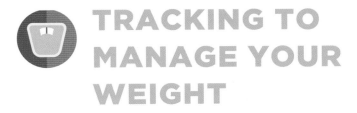

TRACKING TO MANAGE YOUR WEIGHT

To lose, gain, or maintain your weight, it's all about correctly balancing the amount of calories you eat with the amount your body uses through daily living and physical activity. When you eat just as many calories as your body uses, your weight stays the same. When you eat more calories than your body uses, you gain weight. On the other hand, when you eat fewer calories than your body uses,

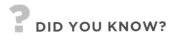

DID YOU KNOW?

One out of every five smartphone owners uses a health app to track or manage their health.

you lose weight. Digitally tracking food and activity helps you balance calories in and calories out so that you can achieve your weight goals.

BUILDING HEALTHY HABITS FOR LOSING WEIGHT

Getting to a healthy weight—and keeping the weight off—means forming healthy habits and sticking with them. Most successful weight-loss programs focus on these lifestyle habits:

- Eat and drink fewer calories ("calories in").
- Be more physically active ("calories out").
- Self-monitor, or be aware of, eating and physical activity behavior.

? WHAT IS A CALORIE?

Calories are the energy supplied by food. Carbohydrates, fats, and protein provide calories. Everyone has different calorie needs. The amount of calories you need depends on your age, sex, physical activity level, height, and weight.

Changing habits can be hard, but using tracking to self-monitor behaviors can help. By tracking your food and physical activity, you will begin to see patterns in your choices. When you see these patterns, they can be easier to change. For example, perhaps you begin to see that you consume a large portion of your daily calories in front of the television most nights or eat bigger portions when dining out with certain friends. Tracking can help you recognize these habits and identify where you can make positive changes.

TRACKING TO MAINTAIN A HEALTHY WEIGHT

Perhaps you have already lost weight, or you just want to stay at your current weight; digital tracking is beneficial for maintainers, too! The National Weight Control Registry studies the eating, exercise, and lifestyle habits of people who have lost weight and kept it off for 1 year or longer. The registry's goal is to find the common strategies of people who maintain their weight loss. The strategies are shared with others to help them achieve the same success. Turns out digital tracking can make most of these weight-loss maintaining habits easier! Here are the seven lifestyle habits of people who maintain their weight loss, and how to use digital tracking to achieve them:

SUCCESSFUL HABIT	WHAT TO DO	HOW TECHNOLOGY CAN HELP
Eat breakfast	Eat breakfast every day. Try on-the-go breakfasts if you are busy, such as a peanut butter and banana sandwich, yogurt and granola in a cup, or a whole-grain cereal bar with a piece of fruit.	Some food log apps alert you to enter your food if you haven't by a certain time of the day, which could remind you to eat breakfast if you missed it. Check the app's settings.
Engage in regular physical activity	Do at least 30 minutes, 5 times a week (150 minutes total), of moderate-intensity physical activity. Start slow and work up to 20 minutes a day if you aren't used to exercising. Check with your doctor before you begin.	Use fitness apps and wearable devices to log your time spent exercising and see how many calories you burn.

SUCCESSFUL HABIT	WHAT TO DO	HOW TECHNOLOGY CAN HELP
Decrease sitting screen time	Limit time sitting in front of the TV and non–work related "screen time" to less than one and a half hours a day (or 10 hours a week).	For extra entertainment, challenge yourself or others on your fitness tracking app. See if you can beat the number of steps you took the day before.
Self-track	Weigh yourself regularly. Track your food intake every day. Log how many minutes you exercise.	Use any self-tracking app, website, or device that you find fun, easy, and interesting!
Follow a healthy eating plan	Aim for 20% to 35% of calories from fat. Look for lower-calorie foods. Choose foods with little added sugar.	Food logs track calories, fat, and sugar for you.
Maintain control over eating habits	Be in charge of your eating habits. Don't eat "just because it's there" or out of emotion.	Some apps let you type in text along with your food entry. If you are bored, hungry, tired, angry, or happy while eating, take note. You may find there are certain times of the day you are more likely to stress-eat.
Resist overeating less healthy foods	Log your food *before* you eat. This makes you think twice before splurging on foods. Use logs to learn portion sizes of high-calorie foods.	Use the "Favorite Foods" list on food trackers to make logging even easier and faster.

Overall, weight-loss maintainers commit to long-term behavior changes—not quick fixes. Food logs and fitness devices can make these important lifestyle changes easy, exciting, and even fun!

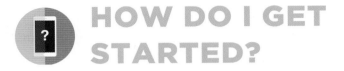

HOW DO I GET STARTED?

You want to start using digital tracking tools. So how do you get started?

You can access digital tools in two ways: through a website or by downloading the app. If you mostly use your computer, you will likely use a website. If you have a smartphone, using an app might be the way to go.

Many people use both. Many tracking tools have both a website version and an app version. For example, you can log your breakfast on the Lose It! app and your lunch from a computer by visiting www.loseit.com.

SIGNING UP ONLINE

To start tracking on a website, you will need to sign up for an account. We are going to use the Lose It! website (www.loseit.com) as an example, but you can use the tracking website you like best. (See Chapter 5 to compare options.)

NOTE:

Steps may be different on the website you choose, but the overall process will be similar.

STEP 1

From the website's homepage, look for the button to sign up. For example, on the Lose It! website, you'll see a button that says "Start Losing It!" You may see "Register," "Get started," or "Create an account" on other websites.

STEP 2

Enter your information. You will need to provide your e-mail address and create a password. Answer the questions to create your personal profile.

STEP 3

When you finish creating your profile, the website will take you to your personal home page where you can track your food, activity, and other health goals.

STEP 4

Remember your log-in information so you can sign in every day.

DOWNLOADING AN APP ON YOUR APPLE iPHONE OR iPAD

STEP 1

Tap "App Store" from your home screen.

STEP 2

If you know what app you want, tap the search magnifying glass at the bottom of the screen. Type the name of the app at the top of the screen. To browse apps, tap "Top Charts" at the bottom of the screen. Then tap "Categories" in the top left corner. Scroll down to "Health & Fitness."

STEP 3

When you've found the app you want, tap on the name.

STEP 4

Tap "Get" and then "Install" to download.

STEP 5

Press the home button to go back to the home screen. Find your app by swiping your finger left or right until you see the app icon. Tap the icon to open.

DOWNLOADING AN APP ON YOUR ANDROID SMARTPHONE OR TABLET

STEP 1

From your home screen, tap the Google Play icon.

STEP 2

If you know what app you want, tap the search magnifying glass and type the name of the app. If you want to browse for apps, tap "Categories" at the top of the screen. Digital health-tracking apps will be under the group called "Health & Fitness."

STEP 3

When you've found the app you want, tap the install button.

STEP 4

After the app is done downloading, find it by tapping the Apps icon or by looking at your home screen.

* NOTE:

Steps may be different on your device, but the overall process will be similar.

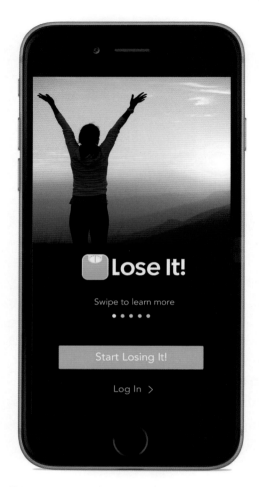

Welcome page for Lose It!, a popular tracking app.
SOURCE: WWW.LOSEIT.COM

REAL-LIFE STORY—PAMELA I.

What do you track?

"I track my food, activity, and water intake by using an app on my smartphone. It took some time to get in the habit of logging. I soon realized my habits, which made it easier over time. I can copy entire meals to another day if I eat the same foods."

Why do you track?

"Tracking lets me know when I'm not eating enough protein or eating too much fat or carbohydrates. I like to track my activities and see how many calories I'm burning. I also want to make sure I'm drinking enough water. If I drink water like I'm supposed to, I feel a lot better."

How often do you track?

"I track my food, water, and activities every day. The more I track, the more I learn about what I'm putting into my body. I can make better choices about what I plan to do or eat."

How does tracking help you?

"If I eat healthy and drink water like I should, my body performs well. Tracking has taught me about portion size, too. Calories add up even if you are eating 3 cups of broccoli!"

CHAPTER 2

WHAT SHOULD I TRACK?

IN 2013 ALONE, there were more than 600 million downloads of health-related apps! With so many different websites, apps, and wearable devices out there, it can be hard to decide what to use and what to track. This chapter will discuss tracking food, fluids, physical activity, weight, and sleep. Some digital tools track all of these things, and others track just some of them. It's up to you what you want to track – you can track several habits, or start out tracking just one or two.

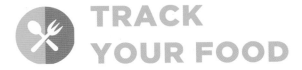

TRACK YOUR FOOD

As you learned in Chapter 1, weight loss occurs when you consume fewer calories than you use. Therefore, knowing how many calories you eat is an important part of managing your weight. It is very common to think we eat less than we actually do, which is where digitally tracking your food can come in handy. Do you know how many calories there are in your morning latte? Your digital food tracker does!

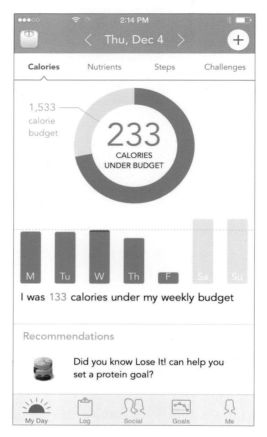

Here's an example of a food-tracking app that counts calories for you. This person has a daily budget of 1,533 calories. Based on what she has already eaten, the app says she can eat 233 more calories for the day.
SOURCE: WWW.LOSEIT.COM

TRACKING CALORIES

Digital trackers take the guesswork out of counting calories. Everyone's calorie needs are different, and digital trackers can help you find your specific daily calorie target. When you set up your account, you will be asked to enter your:

- age,
- sex,
- height,
- weight,
- current physical activity level, and
- weight loss or weight maintenance goal.

The tracker uses this information to calculate a daily calorie target that will help you achieve your goal.

When you enter the food you eat into a digital tracker, it tallies the number of calories for you. You can easily see how close you are to your daily calorie target, and you can use this information to help plan out your meals and snacks. For example, if you eat a higher-calorie breakfast, you'll know to have a lighter lunch or dinner so you don't go over your calorie budget.

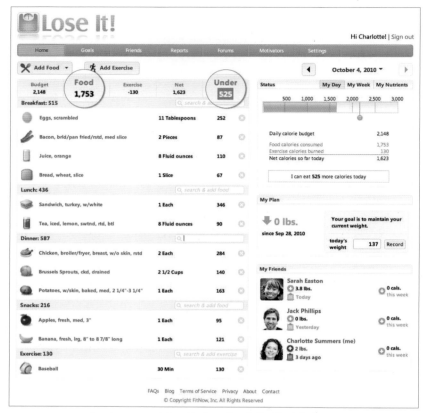

Here is an example from the Lose It! website. Charlotte has entered the foods and beverages and portion sizes for each meal, including snacks. Lose It! has calculated the number of calories in each food. It provides a running total for the day. You can see that Charlotte has eaten 1,753 calories today, 525 calories less than her budgeted amount.
SOURCE: WWW.BLOG.LOSEIT.COM

TRACK YOUR FOOD CHOICES

In addition to calories, most digital food trackers track how much carbohydrate, fat, protein, added sugars, sodium, vitamins, and minerals you eat. It is important to eat an appropriate amount of carbohydrates, fat, and protein every day because each of these nutrients helps the body in different ways. Digital food logs can compare your percentages with a healthy eating goal, so you can see if you're on the right track.

SCAN FOR NUTRITION

Some apps have a bar code scanner! Scan the bar code on the food package and the app automatically finds the food and its nutrition information.

TRACK WHEN YOU EAT

Digital tracking isn't just about what we eat—it's also about paying attention to when we eat. People often eat very differently based on the time of day. Some people eat nothing or very little in the morning and then eat larger amounts of food for lunch or dinner because they are very hungry. Others snack on small amounts of food all day but don't realize how much the calories add up. These types of eating habits may make it hard to stay within your calorie goal. Digital tracking helps you look at your day as a whole and identify where you

A NOTE ABOUT PORTION SIZES

Getting the portion size right is vital to getting accurate results from your tracking tool. It is easy to underestimate the amount of food you eat, and that can really slow reaching your weight and fitness goals. Use measuring cups and spoons or a food scale to measure or weigh your food in order to get the most accurate results.

DID YOU KNOW?

Want to log your lunch but you're not near a computer? Forgot your smartphone at home when heading to work? No problem! Digital trackers are as flexible as you are. Some have apps and websites so you can log on both. Your information will automatically update on both.

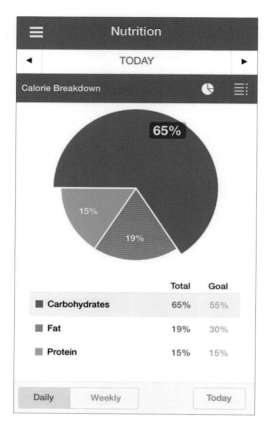

This is a calorie breakdown daily summary from MyFitness Pal. For most healthy adults, experts recommend 55% of our daily calories should come from carbohydrates, 30% from fat, and 15% from protein. Based on her logging, this person has gone over her carbohydrate goal. She has room to eat a little more fat, and she has met her protein goal for the day. SOURCE: WWW.MYFITNESSPAL.COM

might be overdoing it on calories or falling short on nutrients. If you aim to spread your calories evenly throughout the day, you'll find it easier to control your appetite and your weight.

TRACK WHEN YOU DINE OUT

Choosing healthy options at restaurants can be tricky. Some dinner salads have more calories and fat than the entrees! Conveniently, many digital food trackers have restaurant nutrition information, too, which can be helpful when you dine out. Search for the name of the restaurant you are going to, and look up the calories before ordering your meal. Remember to add any drinks, appetizers, desserts, and bread you eat to your food log, too.

PRO TIP: LEARN FROM THE EXPERTS!

"My clients who track are much more aware of what they are eating and how much. When they track the food they eat, they pay attention to portion sizes. They are more likely to make changes in their eating and exercise when they have a record. They are also excited to share their results and show me their progress."

Stephanie Long, RDN, CDE, Woodbury, New Jersey

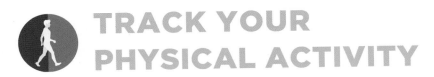

TRACK YOUR PHYSICAL ACTIVITY

Physical activity is an important part of a healthy lifestyle. Physical activity burns calories, which can help you lose or maintain weight. If you are just getting started, aim for at least 150 minutes of moderate-intensity physical activity each week. (That equals 30 minutes, 5 times a week.) Work up to more as you are able—225 to 420 minutes per week is best for weight loss and weight maintenance. This works out to 32–60 minutes a day.

No matter what kind of activity you enjoy—whether it is walking, jogging, biking, swimming, or dancing—you can use digital tools to record your workouts. Just as food trackers help you know how many calories you take in, activity trackers tell you how many calories you burn. Activity trackers also show your progress over time. You can see summaries of your activity level over days, weeks, months, or even years!

Like digital food trackers, digital activity trackers use information about you to recommend how much activity you need to manage your weight. The amount of physical activity needed depends on your:

- age,
- current health and fitness level,
- weight, and
- health goals.

There are different ways to use digital activity trackers. Many people use more than one way. You can:

- enter your activities manually when you complete them, the same way you enter foods into your food tracker;
- open the activity tracker app on your smartphone and carry it with you during your activity, during which it will track and analyze your movements; or
- use a wearable device that automatically sends information about your workout to your computer or smartphone, which you can view later.

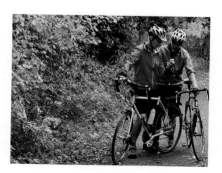

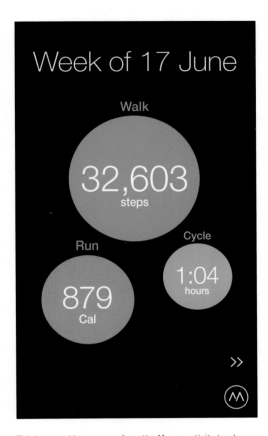

This is a weekly summary from the Moves activity tracker app. It tracks several different types of exercise. In one week, this person has taken 32,603 steps, burned 879 calories running, and cycled for 1 hour and 4 minutes.
SOURCE: WWW.MOVES-APP.COM

TRACK YOUR WORKOUTS

Digital trackers can tell you many things about your workouts. For example, let's say you get in your moderate-intensity physical activity by cycling for 30 minutes 5 days a week. A digital activity tracker can keep track of your time, your distance, your route, and your pace (how fast you move).

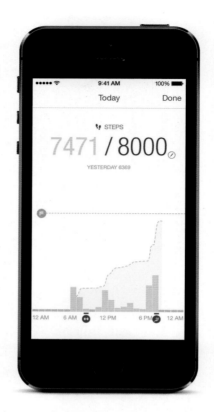

Here's an example of a step counter from the Runtastic app. This person has taken 7,471 steps so far today. The app tells them they take the most steps in the morning, around noon, and in the evening. If they can take more steps midmorning and midafternoon, they will easily meet their personal goal of 8,000 steps per day. The app also tells them how many steps they took yesterday. This person can feel proud that they have already taken more steps today than the day before. SOURCE: WWW.RUNTASTIC.COM

TRACK YOUR ALL-DAY ACTIVITY

Many experts recommend taking more steps during the day for better health. Ever try counting how many steps you take in a day? Thankfully, digital activity trackers use special technology that counts for you!

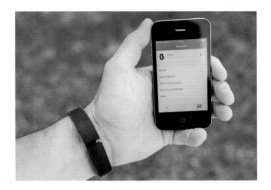

If you have a smartphone, you can download an app that will track your steps throughout the day, but this means you have to be carrying your smartphone with you at all times. You can also wear an activity tracker all day long to make sure you track every step.

Seeing your activity add up can really help motivate you to stay active—which will then naturally improve your fitness and health. See Chapter 5 for tips on finding the right digital physical activity tracker for you.

TRACK YOUR PHYSICAL INACTIVITY

In addition to moving more, sitting less can help you lose weight and keep it off. Spending many hours in front of a TV or computer screen may be harmful to your health. In many studies, physical inactivity has been linked with depression and muscle weakness. Loss of muscle can make daily activities more difficult.

Some wearable devices alert you to stand up if you have been sitting too long. The Apple Watch and Garmin vivofit devices have this feature.

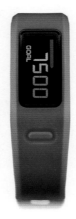

This is a Garmin vivofit wearable activity device. The red bar appears after 1 hour of inactivity and gets longer as you keep sitting. When you stand and move around, the red bar disappears. SOURCE: WWW.GARMIN.COM

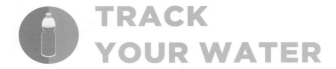

TRACK YOUR WATER

What's the deal with drinking water? Water is necessary for our bodies to work well. Water has many important jobs in our body, such as:

- removing waste;
- protecting our joints and organs;
- keeping our body temperature normal; and
- moving nutrients through the body.

We need to replace the water our bodies lose or we become dehydrated. We may become dehydrated when we are ill, sweating in hot weather, or during physical activity. Drinking water is a great way to stay hydrated. Limit drinks with added sugar because these calories add up quickly and usually don't come with essential nutrients. Try adding fresh fruit, such as lemon wedges or cucumber pieces, to water for a great flavor without the calories.

Drinking water and other no-calorie drinks may help us lose weight, too. Studies have shown that people eat fewer calories at meals when they drink water right before they eat. Another study showed that monitoring how much water you drink also can help with weight loss and weight maintenance.

DIGITAL TOOLS FOR TRACKING WATER

Digital health tracking can also help you stay hydrated. Many digital food trackers let you track how much you drink. There are also some apps that only track fluids, such as Water Your Body. By using these kinds of apps, you can see how much you drink every day and over time. Some trackers estimate how much water you should drink. Some allow you to set reminders about drinking water.

To find a water tracking app, search these phrases in your app store:

- water tracker
- water reminder
- water app

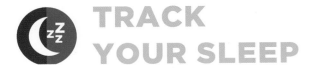 ## TRACK YOUR SLEEP

You may be asking yourself, why is sleep included in a digital weight maintenance book? It's because sleep is vital for health, well-being, and even weight loss! Studies have shown that people who don't get enough sleep are more likely to be overweight. For this reason, it is a good idea to track how many hours you sleep. This is especially true if you think you may be getting too little sleep.

The National Institutes of Health says adults need 7 to 8 hours of sleep every day for good health. Many things can worsen our sleep, such as

- exercising right before bed,
- drinking too much caffeine or alcohol,
- watching a TV or computer screen before bed, or
- eating a large meal before going to bed.

Sleep-tracking technology makes you aware of your habits that may hurt the quality of your sleep. When you are well rested, you have more energy and will more easily meet your fitness goals and improve your health.

There are many digital trackers you can use to improve your sleep. Sleep trackers may include a wearable device that communicates with your computer or smartphone or a device that you place on your bed. Sleep trackers can track:

- how long you sleep,
- quality of sleep,
- sleep cycles, and
- movement during sleep.

Some may include gentle alarms to wake you during your lightest sleep times.

DIGITAL TOOLS FOR TRACKING SLEEP

Just like food and activity trackers, there are several options for apps and devices that track your sleep. Sleep trackers come in three categories: wearable devices worn while sleeping, devices kept in your bed, and apps for your smartphone. Your smartphone is usually placed in the upper corner of your mattress for best results. The following table shows how the different options for tracking sleep are typically used.

SLEEP TRACKING OPTIONS	SLEEP HABITS TRACKED AND FEATURES	HOW TO USE IT
Wearable device	Movement Restfulness Sleep time Quality Silent wake alarm Coaching to improve sleep	Wear on wrist while sleeping Information uploads to smartphone automatically
Bed device	Total sleep time Sleep cycles Awake times Heart rate Snoring Breathing rate Wake alarm	Place in bed on top of mattress Follow manufacturer's instructions for best results
Smartphone apps	Movement Gentle wake alarm Sleep phases Quality Sound tracker (snoring/talking) Resources for better sleep	Place in bed next to pillow Follow app instructions for best results

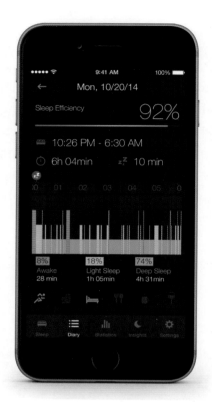

Here is a screen shot from the Sleep Better app by Runtastic on the iPhone. This person had a 92% sleep efficiency.
A higher efficiency means a more restful sleep. This person
did not get 100% sleep efficiency; as you can see, he or
she woke up a few times during the night (shown by the red
bars). Over time, the user will notice what daily habits lead
to a better sleep. SOURCE: WWW.RUNTASTIC.COM

To find a sleep tracking app, search these phrases in your app store:
- sleep tracker
- sleep cycle
- sleep better

TRACK YOUR WEIGHT

Weight tracking is another great feature of many digital trackers. Enter your current weight, and the tracker will graph your weight loss over time. Seeing your progress reminds you of how well you are doing. When you see how well you are doing, you'll want to keep going!

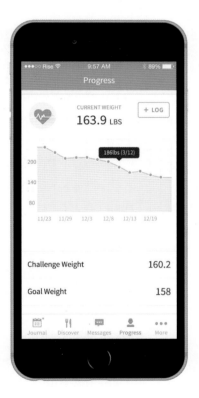

Here is a weight loss graph from Rise's app. This person is 3.7 pounds from reaching his challenge weight and 5.9 pounds from reaching his goal weight. SOURCE: WWW.RISE.US

How often you weigh yourself depends on you. You may choose to weigh in daily, every few days, or weekly. Researchers have found people who weigh themselves every day lose more weight than those who weigh less often. Frequent weighing can be a good tool to monitor your progress.

However, while weighing every day can help you to control your weight, some experts worry it may lead to a harmful obsession with the scale. If you feel discouraged when weighing every day, try once every few days or once a week. Weight loss is slow for some people. If you like seeing bigger changes, this is a good strategy to take.

✚ TIPS FOR WEIGHING IN

For your most accurate weight, weigh yourself:

- on the same day(s) of the week;

- using the same scale;

- when you wake up in the morning, after you've used the restroom; and

- wearing the same clothes (or lack of!)

Try not to go longer than 1 week without weighing yourself. Never weigh yourself more than once a day. There are natural ups and downs to our weight throughout the day. We will always weigh more after a meal than before!

Digital trackers can measure many details of our lives: the food we eat, the exercise we do, the water we drink, our sleep, and our weight. As we have seen, tracking these health habits helps us manage a healthy weight. Remember, maintaining or losing weight is about balancing your calories. Digital tracking can help you see how your calories from food and activity balance out, so you can achieve your weight goals.

REAL-LIFE STORY: BRAD P.

What wearable activity tracker do you use?

"I'm currently wearing a Fitbit Charge. I will get an Apple Watch soon."

What does the device track for you?

"It tracks how many calories I burn, the number of steps I take, and active hours."

Why do you track these things?

"It's a great way to keep a 'check' on me and my activity during the day."

How often do you track and why?

"I try to track daily. Even though it doesn't monitor sleep, I still wear it at night so I don't leave the house without it!"

How do you benefit from tracking and why?

"The tracker is a great motivator. Whatever your goal, 10,000, 15,000, or 20,000 steps a day . . . when evening sets in and you check your device and realize you're short a few steps or. . . a few thousand steps . . . it's a great way to get you moving for one last time before the day ends."

REAL-LIFE STORY: BARBARA J.

What do you track?

"I use a Fitbit and I track steps, sleep, calories eaten, weight, calories burned, miles walked, and active minutes."

Why do you track?

"I track to watch my weight and to increase my exercise. I try to get 10,000 steps in every day. I watch my exercise levels to see how many calories I burn. It also helps me make better food choices."

How often do you track?

"Every day! At the end of the week, I get a weekly report on what I did. I look at my routines to see patterns. Knowing these patterns help me make changes."

How does tracking help you?

"Tracking helps me to see daily and weekly numbers. It helps me make changes and increase daily activity, even if it's taking a few more steps. I have friends who use the Fitbit, too. I can see what they do and they see what I do. We cheer each other on!"

CHAPTER 3

WHY SHOULD I TRACK?

DIGITAL TRACKING IS a great tool for managing your weight for a number of reasons:

- Through self-monitoring, you gain insight into your habits. Counting calories makes the relationship between food, activity, and your weight clear.
- Personal feedback lets you know how you are doing.
- Online communities offer social support that can help keep you going.

Let's take a closer look at each of these benefits.

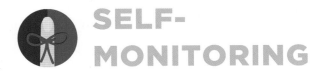

SELF-MONITORING

Self-monitoring helps make you aware of your own behaviors and habits. To improve your health, you may need to change some habits. The first step is to pay attention to, or monitor, your actions and identify the habits that help or hurt your weight and fitness goals. Digital tracking can help.

Self-monitoring makes you aware of things you may do without thinking, which helps you to correct unhealthy habits and develop positive ones instead. For example, Susan tracks her food and notices she eats sugary foods when she watches TV at night. Therefore, she starts eating fruit while watching TV. She feels better the next morning and, over time, she begins to lose weight.

Joe wears a device on his wrist that shows him how many steps he takes in a day. He notices he takes a lot more steps on the days he walks to the grocery store instead of driving. This encourages him to walk to the grocery store more often. Over time, he feels more fit and healthy.

When you use tracking to lose or maintain weight, you will begin to notice things about the foods you eat and the physical activities you do. For example, studies show people tend to under-estimate the number of calories they eat. When you begin tracking, you may be surprised to see how many calories are in your favorite meals! Self-monitoring gives you a chance to think twice before eating something that may not be the best choice. You may not realize how many calories you burn while walking. Tracking the "numbers" makes you aware of how certain foods, activities, and habits affect your health for better or for worse.

The knowledge you get by self-monitoring is a great step toward change. Use digital tracking to become aware of your habits and change them for the better.

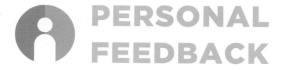

PERSONAL FEEDBACK

A great benefit of many digital tracking tools is personal feed-back, which can come in many forms. Your tracking tool shows you progress over time, encourages you to stick to your goals, and helps you make adjustments to your plan. It can even come from a real coach or dietitian who is live and online!

GET INSPIRED BY YOUR PROGRESS

When you look back at the workouts you have logged or the days you hit your calorie target, it is encouraging to see the progress you have made. This personal feedback helps keep you going.

After each workout, activity trackers show you a summary of your activity. The summary may include how far you went, how fast you went (your pace), how many steps you took, and how many calories you burned. Activity trackers also provide weekly, monthly, and annual summaries. Looking back at this feedback is a great way to reflect on how far you have come. Perhaps you added miles or minutes to your walks. Maybe you increased your speed or strength! Perhaps you have become more regular with your workouts. Noting your achievements helps inspire you to continue your healthy habits.

GET ENCOURAGEMENT

Everyone needs a friendly nudge once in a while. Many digital tracking tools have features that encourage you to stick to your health goals.

For example, it can be hard to form the habit of tracking your food. You may forget, or you simply may not feel like it. If you haven't logged in for a while, expect to get a reminder by e-mail or by a notification on your smartphone. Lose It! lets you set the times you want to be reminded.

Other digital tools provide encouragement when you reach your goal, such as a checkmark or points.

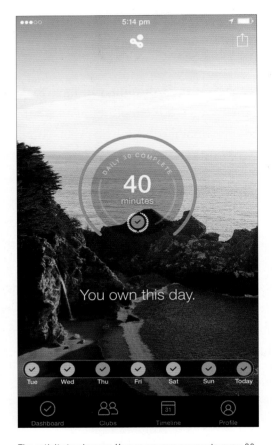

The activity tracker app Human encourages you to move 30 minutes or more every day. It rewards you with a checkmark and an encouraging message each time you accomplish that goal. SOURCE: WWW.HUMAN.CO

GET SPECIFIC

Digital food trackers can give you specific feedback about your daily eating. They can compare your eating habits to general healthy eating guidelines for your age, sex, and activity level. For example, trackers tell you when you eat too much saturated fat, sodium, or cholesterol. They will also tell you if you need to eat more nutrients like fiber, vitamins, and minerals. Digital food logs are one of the easiest ways to make sure you are eating healthfully. You can use this information to identify where you might need to make some changes in your overall food choices.

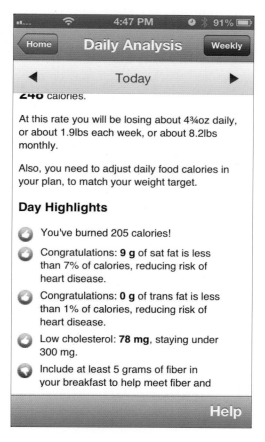

This daily analysis from MyNetDiary shows that the user burned 205 calories doing physical activity. He also stayed within his recommended daily budget for saturated fat, *trans* fat, cholesterol, and sodium (salt). What he needs to work on is eating more fiber at breakfast.
SOURCE: WWW.MYNETDIARY.COM

GET EXPERT HELP

Have a general or specific question about food and health? Many health apps and websites use blogs to answer readers' questions. Some apps and websites even have real, live coaches that can give you personalized feedback. Set goals with these apps, and your coach will help get you there. Ask your coach questions and get new ideas when you feel stuck. Coaches help you make better food choices and suggest new workouts you may enjoy.

One example of a coaching app is Rise (www.rise.us). The coaches are registered dietitian nutritionists (RDNs). When you sign up, you can send photos and messages to your coach and get tips, ideas, and encouragement back.

Personal feedback based on your goals is a great way to stay on track. It helps you understand what you are doing well and what you can improve.

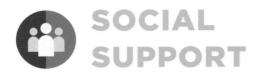

SOCIAL SUPPORT

Weight loss can be challenging, and social support is an important key to success. Many digital tracking tools have an online community full of people who share similar goals. You can communicate with them, and often with nutrition or weight-loss experts too, via message boards, live chats, and blogs. You can also connect with friends so you can follow each other's online activity. Let's take a closer look at some of the ways you can use digital tools to get social support.

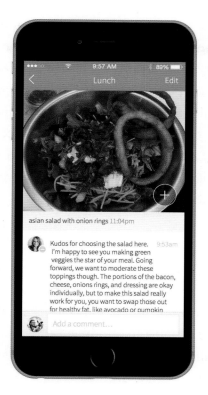

This person used the Rise app to take a photo of his lunch and send it to his RDN coach. She gives him feedback on what he did well and what he can improve upon.
SOURCE: WWW.RISE.US

MESSAGE BOARDS AND FORUMS

Have a question for other users? Use your tracker's message board! Message boards and forums are an easy way to connect with other people when you have a question or need support. Questions range from "what's the healthiest cereal to eat?" to "how do I get through the holidays without gaining weight?" You can ask a question or you can read other people's questions and answers.

Message boards and forums are also great places to find users who have health goals similar to yours. Join groups that share your interests. Examples of special group message boards are Women Over 50, Couch to 5K runners/walkers, and Recipe Sharers. But remember, while message boards and forums are helpful, they are not meant to replace working with a health care professional.

LIVE CHAT

We have talked about using online coaching and coaching apps as a way to get personal feedback. Coaches can also provide support by answering your questions and offering motivation. They can even provide support in a moment of weakness. Craving ice cream at 2:00 a.m.? You might want to look for an app that offers around-the-clock coaching, such as Weight Watchers' 24/7 chat feature, to help resist late-night temptation.

ACTIVITY FEEDS

An activity feed, or news feed, displays your recent activity. For example, if you log a workout or a day's meals, a notification will appear in your activity feed.

If you choose to connect with friends who use the same app or website, their activity appears in your feed, and your activity appears in theirs. What are the benefits? Seeing your friends take action toward their health goals may inspire you to stick to yours. For example, if you see a friend has logged her food for a whole week, you may feel motivated to do the same. You can also post comments to encourage each other.

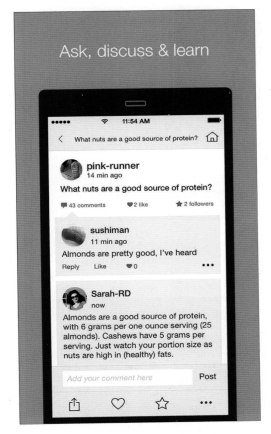

This is a message board from Fooducate's app. Someone wanted to know if nuts are a good source of protein. They got an answer from a fellow user and Sarah, an RDN.
SOURCE: WWW.FOODUCATE.COM

REAL-LIFE STORY: MARCQUIS C.

"I use Runkeeper to track my miles when I run. Friends encourage me to keep going. I like seeing my progress over time. I track every run I do to look back to see how far I've come. It helps me see what I need to work on, too."

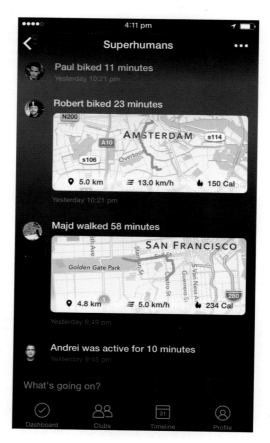

Join a club on the Human activity tracker app! The activity
feed lets you see what other people are doing. They can see
your activity, too, if you choose to share it.
SOURCE: WWW.HUMAN.CO

BLOGS

Many digital trackers offer blogs as another great social support
and education tool. These blogs are regularly updated and feature
short articles on a variety of health-related topics that can help
you to achieve your goals. Topics range from healthy eating tips
and recipes, to ways to decrease stress, to new exercises to try, and

more. Blogs can be read on the digital tracker's app or on their website. For example, MyFitnessPal's blog can be read by visiting www.blog.myfitnesspal.com. Or, go to your tracker's main website and search "blog."

CHALLENGES

There's nothing wrong with a little healthy competition! Many apps allow you to challenge friends to contests. For example, who can take the most steps in one day? But watch out! Others can challenge you just as easily. If you don't want to challenge others, try challenging yourself! See if you can take more steps today than you did yesterday. Can you drink water instead of sugary drinks at least three days a week?

Lose It! offers a variety of challenges you can choose from, depending on your goal, such as weight loss, physical activity, logging, or overall wellness. Choose a challenge that appeals to you. You can participate as an individual or join a team. Don't worry about winning or losing. The important thing is that by participating, you are improving your health.

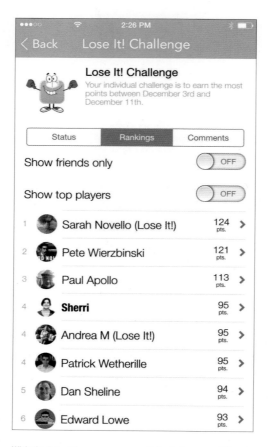

With the Lose It! app, you can participate in many different challenges. In this challenge, the aim is to earn more points than others in the challenge. Users earn points by logging. The more they track their food and exercise, the more points they earn! SOURCE: WWW.LOSEIT.COM

PRO TIP: LEARN FROM THE EXPERTS!

What are the most common habits you encourage your clients/patients to track and why?

"I ask my clients to track what they eat, drink, and [do for] physical activity, as well as how they feel or their thoughts (I feel full, irritated, tired, anxious, hungry, and so on). Tracking allows for a deeper understanding of nutrition and what is necessary for a healthy lifestyle."

What benefits do you see in your clients/patients who do track vs those who don't?

"Tracking puts into perspective how much they eat and drink. People who don't track any behaviors tend to have little overall knowledge of their habits. Tracking adds accountability while also being a great teaching tool. People also begin to understand the connection between energy level, how they feel, and how important nutrition is."

What are the most common apps, websites, or devices your clients/patients use? What do they like about them?

"The most user-friendly apps that my clients have shared with me are Spark People, MyFitnessPal, USDA SuperTracker, and Recovery Record."

Monique Richard, MS, RDN, LDN
Johnson City, Tennessee

CHAPTER 4

HOW DO I GET THE MOST FROM TRACKING?

SHOULD I LOG every meal I eat? How often should I weigh myself? Is it best to track in the morning or the evening? What if I ate something I regret? Should I still track it? All these questions are important to successful tracking.

Successful tracking must include these three things:

- honesty,
- consistency, and
- timing.

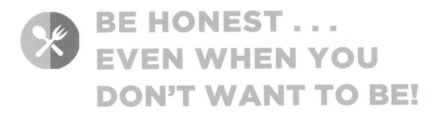

BE HONEST . . . EVEN WHEN YOU DON'T WANT TO BE!

Successful food tracking depends on being honest about what and how much we eat. If we underreport what we eat or overreport our exercise, we may not reach our health goals.

Once in a while, we all do things we regret. It's tempting to not log foods that might put us over our daily calorie budget. However, whether you log the food or not, it still happened. Be honest and forgiving with yourself. Log, learn from the experience, and move on. The simple act of logging makes you more aware of what you're eating and of your activity level.

BE CONSISTENT

Should you track every day? What if you miss logging a meal? How often you track depends on you. Experts have conducted studies to see if constant tracking affects weight loss. In one study, researchers noticed people who logged their food one or two times a week lost less weight than people who logged their food every day. Overall, researchers found regular, everyday tracking leads to:

- losing more weight and keeping it off,
- getting more physical activity,
- eating more fruits and vegetables, and
- drinking more water.

Don't worry if you occasionally forget to track or need to take a short break. Digital tracking will always be there when you choose to start again.

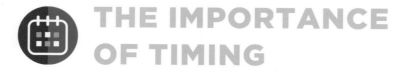

THE IMPORTANCE OF TIMING

If too much time goes by between eating and logging, you may forget what or how much you ate and drank. If your logs are not accurate, then you won't be able to tell if you stayed within your calorie budget for the day. Therefore, experts say the best time for a person to track their food intake is right before or after they eat, when food is on their mind.

Some people find it helpful to enter their food before they eat. It helps them stay within their calorie range for the day and make better food choices. Imagine this: You go to the cafeteria to get lunch. Your choices are meat lasagna or baked salmon. You look up the nutrition information on your food tracking app. Which meal would you choose?

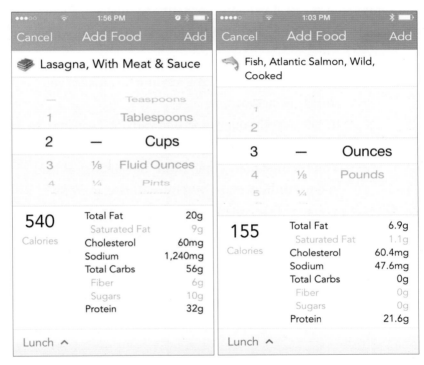

SOURCE: LOSE IT! APP

You would likely choose salmon instead of lasagna. When choosing salmon, you would eat fewer calories and less total fat, saturated fat, and sodium. Remember to change the serving size of the salmon if you eat more than 3 oz before adding it to your food log.

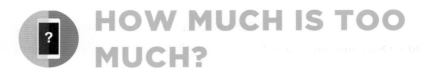

HOW MUCH IS TOO MUCH?

While most people find tracking to be a helpful way to reach their goals, for some, it can stop being a benefit and, instead, become an obstacle. Here are some signs that tracking is interfering with your health goals:

- You don't enjoy tracking anymore. It makes you uneasy or nervous.
- It "takes over" your eating, and you don't feel in control.
- You become preoccupied with how many calories you eat or how many you burn during exercise.
- You may fear certain foods. You change your eating or exercise habits for the worse, not better, by cutting too many calories or exercising too much.

If you notice any of these signs, it's okay to take a break from tracking. Talk to your doctor or RDN about digital tools that can help you achieve your health goals without having to count calories.

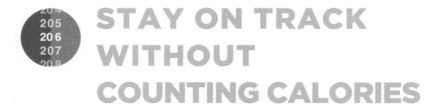

STAY ON TRACK WITHOUT COUNTING CALORIES

Some people don't like counting calories, but they can still track! Digital tracking apps that don't log calories can still help you make healthy food choices. One option is called YouFood. With this app, take photos of your meals, snacks, drinks, and whatever you do to stay healthy. Follow others on their health journey and be inspired. Set your own eating, exercise, and lifestyle goals.

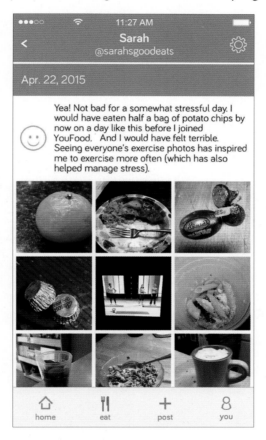

This is a user's daily photos from the YouFood app. She took photos of what she ate and drank during the day. She even took a photo of the exercise video she did! In her comments for the day, the user said using the app helped her stay on track and not eat out of stress. SOURCE: WWW.TWOGRAND.COM

PRO TIP: LEARN FROM THE EXPERTS!

What habits do you encourage your clients to track and why?

"I ask my clients to track food intake, steps, fluid, weight, and sleep. If they aren't ready to track all of this at once, I start them with tracking their food. Using an online tracking tool gives instant feedback. They immediately see how the choices they make impact their overall health (and choices for the rest of the day)! It's like having a dietitian in their back pocket!"

How often do you encourage your clients to track and why?

"I encourage daily nutrition and activity tracking. I ask them to weigh weekly. It's easier to address a small weight gain over 1 week than a 5- or 10-pound weight gain over a month."

What benefits do you see in your clients/patients who do track vs those who don't?

"I did a study that showed daily logging with digital tracking technology led to more weight loss than for those who don't track. I also find people who track learn more about nutrition by paying attention to the foods they eat."

What are the most common apps, websites, or devices your clients use? What do they like about them?

- "MyFitnessPal has a large food database. It's user friendly if they can find the foods they are eating. It has a bar code scanner that people like to use."
- "Fitbits are reliable and their price points can fit most budgets. There's a great social support built in to encourage each other. It accurately tracks steps and links to food logging apps and websites."

Meghann Featherstun, MS, RDN, LD
Shaker Heights, Ohio

REAL-LIFE STORY: CRISTY W.

What do you track?

"I track my calories and my activity levels. I log how many steps I take and how far I walk. I also track how much water I drink. I use the app Lose It!"

Why do you track?

"I track for several reasons:

- to hold myself accountable for my actions and habits,
- to keep track of what I'm eating (good and bad) and my progress, and
- to help with weight loss."

How often do you track?

"I track every day. I do it every day to keep me focused and on track!"

How does tracking help you?

"Tracking helps me make healthy lifestyle changes. I actually see how much or how little activity I am doing. It also helps me 'see' my weight loss progress."

You just started tracking. What keeps you going?

"I keep tracking because of the weight loss I've already seen. I get inspiring messages from other members that keep me going. I also compete in challenges with other members. A challenge that I am doing now is logging in and tracking at least once a day for an entire month. I'm in first place!"

CHAPTER 5

HOW DO I CHOOSE THE RIGHT DIGITAL TOOLS?

READY TO GO digital? There are tens of thousands of health and fitness apps available, and dozens of wearable devices, too. How do you know which digital tools are right for you? This chapter describes the most popular digital health and fitness tools to help you choose. The apps, websites, and tracking devices described in this chapter were chosen based on user reviews and popularity. Many more options exist. You can try searching the app store for what you need or ask your friends if they use health trackers and try theirs.

To choose the tools that are right for you, think about your goals. Do you want to:

- eat healthier,
- become more physically fit,
- sleep better,
- drink more water, or
- find support?

Think about what kind of technology you will use to access these tools, such as your desktop computer or your mobile phone. Also consider if you are willing to spend money on these tools. Many are free, but some come at a cost.

The key to choosing any digital health tool is finding one that helps you reach your goals. Try one for a few days to see if you like it. If not, don't give up! Keep looking until you find the tool that works for you.

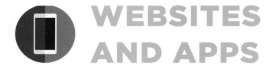

WEBSITES AND APPS

The table below compares the most popular digital dieting websites and apps. See which ones have the features that interest you. Then take a look at the detailed information about each tool to help you decide which one is right for you. You may find you would like to use more than one, and that's OK. Many people do!

DIGITAL DIETING TOOLS: WEBSITES AND APPS OVERVIEW[a]

TOOL	FOOD TRACKER	PHYSICAL ACTIVITY TRACKER	COMMUNITY[b]	COACHING[c]	SLEEP TRACKER	WATER TRACKER	WEB OR MOBILE	COST
Argus	✓	✓	✓		✓	✓	Mobile	Free
Endomondo		✓	✓				Both	Free
Fooducate	✓		✓	✓		✓	Both	Free
Google Fit		✓					Both	Free
Human		✓	✓				Mobile	
Lose It!	✓	✓	✓			✓	Both	Basic: free Premium: $
Lume Wellness	✓	✓	✓		✓	✓	Mobile	Basic: free 42 Day Nutrition Challenge: $
Moves		✓					Mobile	Free
MyDietitian	✓	✓	✓			✓	Mobile	Free

TOOL	FOOD TRACKER	PHYSICAL ACTIVITY TRACKER	COMMUNITY[b]	COACHING[c]	SLEEP TRACKER	WATER TRACKER	WEB OR MOBILE	COST
MyFitnessPal	✓	✓	✓			✓	Both	Basic: free Premium: $
MyNetDiary	✓	✓	✓	✓		✓	Both	Basic: free Premium: $
MyPlate Calorie Tracker	✓	✓	✓			✓	Both	Basic: free Premium: $
Rise	✓			✓			Mobile	Basic: free Premium: $
YouFood	✓		✓			✓	Mobile	Free
USDA SuperTracker	✓	✓				✓	Web	Free

[a] Mention of product names in this publication does not constitute endorsement by the authors or the Academy of Nutrition and Dietetics. Information was accurate at time of publication.

[b] Includes one or a combination of features that help users connect with one another, such as message boards, activity feeds, blogs, or group challenges.

[c] Includes professional services by a professional, such as an RDN or a certified personal trainer.

COMPREHENSIVE DIGITAL TRACKING TOOLS

The digital tools below allow users to track both food and physical activity. Other notable features are listed as well, including different ways they provide social support. Note that app features may change as updates become available.

ARGUS

Platform(s)	Mobile: Apple and Android
Cost	Free
Food tracker	Allows user to take and upload photos of meals and snacks Doesn't count calories Tracks how much water you drink
Physical activity tracker	Counts daily steps Maps exercise using global positioning system (GPS) Tracks calories burned during the day and while exercising Provides voice coaching during exercise
Social support	Can challenge friends to exercise more Comment on friends' activities and progress
Other features	Sets daily goals for steps, sleep, and hydration Measures sleep cycles for better rest Easy to use with wearable devices and other health apps Provides snapshot of daily activity and progress

LOSE IT!

Platform(s)	Online: www.loseit.com Mobile: Apple, Android, Nook, and Kindle
Cost	Basic: free Premium: $39.99 per year
Food tracker	Provides validated nutrition information about thousands of restaurant, grocery store, and brand-name foods Allows user to input recipes and share them with others Has bar code scanner for packaged foods
Physical activity tracker	Features large exercise database Saves frequent exercises
Social support	See friends' progress on activity feed Receive helpful reminders to track Join health and fitness challenges against other users Connect with friends, family, and people with similar health goals Read blogs on healthy eating and fitness

LUME WELLNESS

Platform(s)	Mobile: Apple
Cost	Basic: Free 42 Day Nutrition Challenge: $19.99
Food tracker	Tracks food groups eaten instead of calories Logs water intake
Physical activity tracker	Automatically tracks steps while walking or running See calories burned and miles traveled
Social support	Post activity to Facebook for encouragement from your friends
Other features	Set your own goals Meditation timer Track mood and energy levels Record weight changes

MYDIETITIAN

Platform(s)	Online: www.mydietitian.com Mobile: Apple and Android
Cost	$79.99 per month Premium Plus: $109 per month
Food tracker	Personal RDN available 7 days a week Provides feedback and recommendations based on user's daily diet Allows user to upload pictures of meals, along with more detailed information
Physical activity tracker	User can input daily physical activity for RDN to acknowledge when reviewing daily diet
Social support	Daily summary from personal RDN Can receive feedback via text, voicemail, or video clip
Other features	Helps user track sleep and stress levels

MYFITNESSPAL

Platform(s)	Online: www.myfitnesspal.com Mobile: Apple, BlackBerry, Windows, and Android
Cost	Basic: free Premium: $9.99 per month; $49.99 per year
Food tracker	Allows user to input recipes Saves favorite foods and meals Has bar code scanner for packaged foods Features a large food database
Physical activity tracker	Counts daily steps Features large exercise database
Social support	Participate in community message boards Read daily updates to blogs See friends' progress on activity feed Receive helpful reminders to track
Other features	Connects with wearable devices and fitness apps. Work out with a fitness app and your data will show up in MyFitnessPal.

MYNETDIARY

Platform(s)	Online: www.mynetdiary.com Mobile: Apple, Blackberry, and Android

Cost	Website membership options:
	    PRO: $9 for one month; $24 for 3 months; $42 for 6 months; $60 per year
	App options:
	    Basic: free
	    PRO: $3.99

Food tracker	Features a large food database Saves favorite foods Has bar code scanner for packaged foods Helps user make healthier choices by "grading" foods Ability to enter special foods and your own recipes

Physical activity tracker	Features more than 500 activities and exercises Allows user to enter custom exercises Connects with other fitness apps and wearable devices
Social support	Join community forums and blog with an RDN Connect with friends, share news and comments Link diary with Twitter account
Other features	Users can ask an RDN for personal advice

MYPLATE CALORIE TRACKER

Platform(s)	Online: www.livestrong.com/myplate Mobile: Apple and Android
Cost	Basic: free Gold membership: $9.99 for one month; $30 for 6 months; $45 per year
Food tracker	Uses easy "one-click" tracking Creates personalized meal plans with recipes and shopping lists with Gold membership Features daily nutrition charts, graphs, and goals Tracks how much water you drink
Physical activity tracker	Features guided, high-intensity workout plans with Gold membership Allows user to enter custom exercises
Social support	Receive daily motivations and tips Participate in community forums and blogs Join private support group with membership
Other features	Ability to print data to show your doctor or RDN Reminders to log food

USDA SUPERTRACKER

Platform(s)	Online: www.supertracker.usda.gov
Cost	Free
Food tracker	Saves favorite foods list Creates sample meal plans based on calorie goal Generates list of foods normally eaten together, like cereal and milk Allows user to input recipes
Physical activity tracker	Saves favorite exercises Tracks weekly total minutes of activity
Social support	Can set goals for weight, physical activity, calories, food groups, and nutrients Receive tips from My Coach Center based on your goals
Other features	Food-A-Pedia compares more than 8,000 foods side by side Ability to print or e-mail data to show your doctor or RDN

DIGITAL FOOD AND NUTRITION TOOLS

These digital food and nutrition tools can help you eat better. They offer features like one-on-one coaching, assigning grades to your favorite foods, and photo logging. Each tool can help you manage your weight by encouraging you to eat better and be more active.

FOODUCATE

Platform(s)	Website: www.fooducate.com
Cost	Free
Features	Ability to track quality of calories, not just quantity A bar code scanner so user can quickly find nutrition information about food while grocery shopping Grading system to determine how healthy foods are Suggestions for healthier options in place of less-healthy foods Ability to ask questions and get feedback from the community Daily health tips and recipes

RISE

Platform(s)	Mobile: Apple devices
Cost	Three membership options: Weekly for $19; monthly for $48; 3 months for $120
Features	Advice from RDNs No calorie counting: send photos of what you eat to your coach Interaction with coaches specializing in weight loss, diabetes, sports nutrition, women's health, men's health, heart heath, allergies, and more Ability to message your coach whenever you need them

YOUFOOD

Platform(s)	Mobile: Apple and Android devices
Cost	Free
Features	No calorie counting; instead, take photos of meals, snacks, and exercise, and see a visual history of your eating habits Ability to find people to follow based on goals, lifestyle, and food preferences—and then be inspired by their success!

DIGITAL PHYSICAL ACTIVITY TOOLS

You can download these apps to your smartphone and use them to record your physical activity. Many people enjoy the social part of these apps. Find friends and see how active they are. Challenge them to a physical activity competition and watch the calories burn away!

ENDOMONDO

Platform(s)	Website: www.endomondo.com Mobile: Apple, Android, Blackberry, and Windows Phone
Cost	Basic: free Premium: $5.99 per month; $29.99 per year
Physical activity tracker	Uses GPS to track your physical activity Shows duration, speed, distance, and calories during and after exercise Keeps a full exercise log with workout history
Social support	Send and get pep talks from friends View a newsfeed and comment on friends' progress Set an exercise goal and the app will cheer you on! Join fitness challenges
Other features	Audio feedback during exercise Ability to add photos of workouts Easy to use with wearable devices Premium subscription offers training plans

GOOGLE FIT

Platform(s)	Website: www.google.com/fit Mobile: Android
Cost	Free
Physical activity tracker	Tracks, measures, and stores fitness information Sets goals for your fitness level Shows daily activities and how long you do them Compares activity over time so you can see your improvement
Social support	None
Other features	Can see data from other fitness apps and wearable devices if using multiple apps

HUMAN

Platform(s)	Mobile: Apple and Android devices
Cost	Free
Physical activity tracker	Automatically tracks movement while walking, running, and biking Counts active minutes while moving indoors Provides daily overview of calories burned Shows a quick view of daily activity
Social support	Create or join a club Share progress with friends in your club Receive alerts when you have been inactive
Other features	Get a check mark for at least 30 minutes of movement

MOVES

Platform(s)	Mobile: Apple and Android devices
Cost	Free
Physical activity tracker	Automatically tracks more than 60 types of exercise Provides a daily timeline view of physical activity Counts steps taken throughout the day Uses GPS to track distance
Social support	None
Other features	Recognizes places in your daily life Plots your route on a map

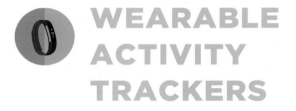

WEARABLE ACTIVITY TRACKERS

Wearable activity trackers are devices you wear on the body (usually the wrist). They monitor your movement and physical activity during the day. You may already be familiar with pedometers, the simple clip-on devices that track your steps. In recent years, wearable activity trackers have come a long way. They include a wide variety of features that can help you achieve your health goals. They send information to a website or app, where you can see your progress over time.

SHOPPING GUIDE: FIND THE FEATURES THAT SUPPORT YOUR GOALS

Let's take a look at features you are likely to find in many of the wearable devices on the market. Which features interest you? Talk to your RDN about the features that may best support your health goals.

- Step counter: Devices with a step counter can count the number of steps you take. To improve or maintain health, many people work up to taking 10,000 steps per day.
- Sleep tracker: Curious to see how well you sleep at night? Some wearable devices track your movement and restfulness when worn while sleeping. View your sleep information on your smartphone the next day.
- Heart-rate monitor: Wearable devices that measure your heart rate more accurately measure the calories you burn at rest and during exercise.
- GPS: Some wearable devices use GPS to know how far you walk and the distance you travel when doing other exercises. Others contain a device called an accelerometer. GPS is usually more accurate.
- Compatibility: Many devices sync with popular websites and apps. This allows you to store all your tracking data in one spot. The device will send information about your activity to your favorite digital tracker. For example, Fitbit lets users link their devices with Lose It!, MyFitnessPal, and many other health apps.

The table below will help you compare some of the more popular wearable devices on the market. Refer to product websites for up-to-date information on features, availability, and cost.

DIGITAL DIETING TOOLS: WEARABLE-DEVICES OVERVIEW[a]

TOOL	STEP COUNTER	ACTIVE MINUTES	CALORIES BURNED	SLEEP TRACKER	INACTIVITY TRACKER	HEART RATE MONITOR	USES GPS	DEVICE COMPATABILITY
Apple Watch	✓	✓	✓		✓	✓	✓	Apple
Basis Peak	✓	✓	✓	✓		✓	✓	Apple & Android
Fitbit Flex	✓	✓	✓	✓				Apple, Android, & Windows
Fitbit Charge HR	✓	✓	✓	✓		✓		Apple, Android, & Windows
Garmin Vivofit 2	✓	✓	✓	✓	✓			Apple & Android
Jawbone UP2	✓	✓	✓	✓	✓			Apple & Android
Jawbone UP Move	✓	✓	✓	✓				Apple & Android
Microsoft Band	✓	✓	✓	✓		✓	✓	Apple, Android, & Windows
Mio Fuse	✓	✓	✓			✓		Apple & Android
Misfit Shine	✓	✓	✓	✓				Apple, Android, & Windows
Soleus GO!	✓	✓	✓	✓	✓			Apple & Android
Withings Pulse O2	✓	✓	✓	✓		✓		Apple & Android

[a] Mention of product names in this publication does not constitute endorsement by the authors or the Academy of Nutrition and Dietetics. Information was accurate at time of publication.

REVIEWS AND UPDATED INFORMATION

Technology moves very fast, and health-tracking websites, apps, and fitness devices can change just as quickly. It's important to stay up to date on the latest products out there, but how? Here are some websites that will help keep you posted on new products and changes to older ones:

- *Food & Nutrition Magazine* app reviews
  - The latest health apps reviewed by food and nutrition experts
  - www.FoodAndNutrition.org/Nutrition-Apps
- MobiHealth News
  - Daily news feed on mobile health news and research, including product updates
  - www.mobihealthnews.com
- iMedicalApps by MedPage Today
  - Physician-edited, unbiased reviews and updates on mobile medical technology
  - www.imedicalapps.com
- Wareable.com
  - News and reviews on the latest wearable devices for fitness tracking and more
  - http://www.wareable.com/fitness-trackers

CHAPTER 6

TAKE YOUR TRACKING TO THE NEXT LEVEL

YOU'VE DONE A great job tracking your food and physical activity! You worked hard to change your habits and even had fun along the way. Now you are ready to take your digital tracking to the next level. Working with a registered dietitian nutritionist (RDN) as you digitally track can help you achieve your goals faster and easier. This chapter will discuss why you should consider working with an RDN and what you can expect to track while working with your RDN.

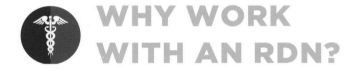

WHY WORK WITH AN RDN?

RDNs are experts in food and nutrition. They became experts through high-level education and supervised experience helping people eat better. An RDN is trained to give you the best and most accurate food and nutrition information. They create an eating plan just for you. There are no one-size-fits-all diets with RDNs!

RDNs have met the following criteria to earn the RDN credential:

- earned a minimum of a bachelor's degree in dietetics, human nutrition, etc, at a US regionally accredited university or college
- completed a supervised practice program at a health care facility, community agency, or a food-service corporation

- passed a national examination and are maintaining registration with continuing professional education

RDNs are trained to teach you about healthy eating. They are also trained to help you make important lifestyle changes. Learning to eat smarter, sort through nutrition misinformation, read food labels, and cook healthy recipes are just some of the skills you will gain from working with an RDN. RDNs also know how to help you eat if you have health conditions like diabetes, high blood pressure, stomach problems, food allergies or intolerances, or heart disease. Additionally, RDNs will make sure you avoid nutrient deficiencies while you are changing your eating habits.

Studies have been done to see how effective RDNs are when it comes to helping people lose weight. Turns out, they are very effective! A study done in 2013 showed that people who were in a weight-loss program while working with RDNs lost more weight and were more physically active compared to those who participated in the program on their own without any outside support. Getting guidance from a RDN is linked to better weight-loss success.

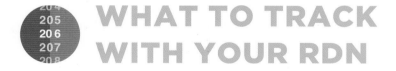 # WHAT TO TRACK WITH YOUR RDN

Using digital tracking tools with your RDN is fun, easy, and helpful. Your RDN will help you learn your habits—good or bad. RDNs will also help you understand why some behaviors are important to change. But first, you need to track your routines honestly and completely. Here is a list of basic habits your RDN may ask you to track:

- what foods you eat and how much
- how much water or other liquids you drink
- what exercises you do and for how long
- your weight (ask your RDN how often you should weigh yourself)

To help even more, your RDN may ask you to track these habits, too:

- when you eat your meals and snacks
- how you feel when you eat (hungry, full, bored, sad)
- where you eat (at the dinner table, in the car, at your desk)
- how well you sleep at night (by using a sleep tracking app)
- the number of steps you take each day

This is a sample of what it may look like when you track with a RDN. Notice the amount of food eaten is listed. It's important to be specific. For example, this person included what he put in their coffee and how his chicken was prepared.

WHEN I ATE	WHAT I ATE	WHERE I ATE	HOW I FELT
Breakfast: 8:15 a.m.	1 slice whole-wheat toast 1 tbsp natural peanut butter 1 medium banana 8 oz coffee with 2 tbsp creamer and 2 tsp sugar	At kitchen table	Rushed to eat before I left for work
Morning snack: 11:00 a.m.	1/3 cup raw almonds	At desk	Hungry; ready for my morning snack

WHEN I ATE	WHAT I ATE	WHERE I ATE	HOW I FELT
Lunch: **12:30 p.m.**	2 cups fresh spinach 3 oz grilled boneless, skinless chicken breast 1 cup whole strawberries 2 tbsp light balsamic vinaigrette dressing 12 oz can diet cola	In cafeteria with coworkers	Not hungry or full; I tried to eat slowly
Afternoon snack: **4:00 p.m.**	Bag of chips	At desk	Stressed at work. I couldn't resist the temptation of the vending machine.
Dinner: **7:00 p.m.**	3/4 cup lentil stew with carrots and vegetables 1/2 cup brown rice	At kitchen table with family	Happy to eat dinner with my family
Nighttime snack: **9:00 p.m.**	1 cup mango	In front of TV	Relaxed

Water	32 oz of water during the day
Physical activity	10-minute walk during my morning break at work Walked 2 miles after dinner
Feelings/ mood	Feeling very hungry on my way home from work Energized and motivated after evening walk

After tracking with his RDN, he learned he often eats at work due to stress. His RDN suggested bringing a healthier snack to eat, such as hummus and raw vegetables, instead of going to the vending machine. His RDN also recommended he eat his morning snack earlier than 11:00 a.m. so he doesn't get too hungry.

USING DIGITAL TRACKING TOOLS WITH YOUR RDN

Recording habits for your RDN is easier when you use digital tracking tools. Using a smartphone, tablet, or your computer is an easy and fast way to connect with your RDN. You won't have to wait until your next session to ask a question. You feel more engaged in your own health and well-being—and you don't even have to pick up the phone! With more and more people preferring to use cell phones instead of landline phones, and many even preferring to send text messages rather than making voice calls, using an app's messaging system should feel easy and natural. And staying in touch and accountable to your RDN will lead to more success.

If you are already working with an RDN, ask if using digital tracking tools is right for you. Because many food and fitness apps take different guidelines into consideration or focus on different aspects of healthy eating and activity, your RDN can help you choose which app is right for you. To find a "virtual" RDN, see Chapter 5 of this book and use the apps and websites that have a coaching* feature.

Surveys show health apps are used more if recommended by or connected to a physician. The same can possibly be said when the app is linked to an RDN. When your RDN asks you to use a digital tracking tool, it is a great opportunity to engage in your health and well-being.

Coaches may or may not be RDNs. Check the app before downloading.

? WHERE DO I FIND AN RDN TO WORK WITH?

Visit www.eatright.org and click "Find an Expert."

Call your medical insurance company and ask for a list of RDNs in your area.

Ask your primary care provider for a referral.

SOURCES

SOURCES

INTRODUCTION

Burke LE, Wang J, Sevick MA. Self-monitoring in weight loss: a systematic review of the literature. *J Am Diet Assoc.* 2011;111(1):92-102.

Centers for Disease Control and Prevention (CDC). Finding a balance. CDC Division of Nutrition, Physical Activity, and Obesity website. http://www.cdc.gov/healthyweight/calories/index.html. Updated May 15, 2015. Accessed September 30, 2015.

Centers for Disease Control and Prevention (CDC). Body mass index. CDC Division of Nutrition, Physical Activity, and Obesity website. http://www.cdc.gov/healthyweight/assessing/bmi/. Updated May 15, 2015. Accessed June 9, 2015.

Fox S, Duggan M. Tracking for health. Pew Research Center website. http://pewinternet.org/Reports/2013/Tracking-for-Health. Published January 28, 2013. Accessed March 12, 2015.

Kumar S, Nilsen WJ, Abernethy A, et al. Mobile health technology evaluation: the mHealth evidence workshop. *Am J Prev Med.* 2013;45(2):228-236.

CHAPTER 1

Fox S, Duggan M. Tracking for health. Pew Research Center website. http://pewinternet.org/Reports/2013/Tracking-for-Health. Published January 28, 2013. Accessed March 12, 2015.

Gilmore LA, Duhe AF, Frost EA, Redman LM. The technology boom: a new era in obesity management. *J Diabetes Sci and Tech.* 2014;8(3):596-608.

Physical Activity Guidelines Advisory Committee. *Physical Activity Guidelines Advisory Committee report, 2008.* Washington, DC: US Department of Health and Human Services, 2008.

Sage S. How to install Android apps. Android Central website. http://www.androidcentral.com/android-apps-install. Published May 2, 2011. Accessed April 7, 2015.

Thomas JG, Bond DS, Phelan S, Hill JO, Wing RR. Weight-loss maintenance for 10 years in the National Weight Control Registry. *Am J Prev Med.* 2014;46(1):17-23.

US Department of Agriculture and US Department of Health and Human Services. *Dietary Guidelines for Americans, 2010.* 7th ed. Washington, DC: US Government Printing Office; 2010.

Yu Z, Sealy-Potts C, Rodriguez J. Dietary Self-monitoring in weight management: current evidence on efficacy and adherence[published online ahead of print May 29, 2015]. *J Acad Nutr Diet.* doi:10.1016/j.jand.2015.04.005.

CHAPTER 2

Centers for Disease Control and Prevention. Finding a balance. CDC Division of Nutrition, Physical Activity, and Obesity website. http://www.cdc.gov/healthyweight/calories/. Updated May 15, 2015. Accessed September 30, 2015.

Centers for Disease Control and Prevention. Water: meeting your daily fluid needs. http://www.cdc.gov/healthywater/drinking/nutrition/ Accessed April 2, 2015.

Cunningham E. What impact does water consumption have on weight loss or weight loss maintenance? *J Acad Nutr Diet.* 2014;114(12):2084.

Donnelly JE, Blair SN, Jakicic JM, Manore MM, Rankin JW, Smith BK. Appropriate physical activity interventions for weight loss and prevention of weight regain for adults. *Med Sci Sports Exerc.* 2009;41(2):459-469.

Kuehn BM. Is there an app to solve app overload? *JAMA.* 2015;313(14):1405-1407.

National Institutes of Health. How much sleep is enough? National Heart, Lung, and Blood Institute website. http://www.nhlbi.nih.gov/health/health-topics/topics/sdd/how-much. Updated February 22, 2012. Accessed June 18, 2015.

National Sleep Foundation. Diet, exercise and sleep. National Sleep Foundation website. http://sleepfoundation.org/sleep-topics/diet-exercise-and-sleep?page=0%2C2. Published December 2009. Accessed April 9, 2015.

Steinberg DM, Bennett GG, Askew S, Tate DF. Weighing every day matters: daily weighing improves weight loss and adoption of weight control behaviors. *J Acad Nutr Diet.* 2015;115(4):511-518.

Tudor-Locke C, Hatano Y, Pangrazi RP, Kang M. Revisiting "how many steps are enough?" *Med Sci Sports Exerc.* 2008;40(7S):S537-S543.

CHAPTER 3

Burke LE, Wang J, Sevick MA. Self-monitoring in weight loss: a systematic review of the literature. J Am Diet Assoc. 2011; 111:92-102.

Conroy MB, Yang K, Elci OU, et al. Physical activity self-monitoring and weight loss: 6-month results of the SMART trial. *Med Sci Sports Exerc.* 2011;43(8):1568-1574.